BAD MEDICINE

William Campbell Douglass, MD

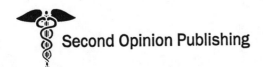

Second Opinion Publishing

Copyright © 1994

by

William Campbell Douglass, M.D.

Additional copies of this book may be purchased from Second Opinion Publishing for $8.95. Second Opinion Publishing also publishes Dr. Douglass's monthly "contrary opinion" medical newsletter, *Second Opinion*. An introductory subscription to *Second Opinion* is $49 for 1 year, $89 for 2 years. Contact *Second Opinion*, Post Office Box 467939, Atlanta, Georgia 31146-7939. Or call 1-800-728-2288.

ISBN 1-885236-00-X

Cover design by Elizabeth Bame

For information regarding this book, call or write:

Second Opinion Publishing, Inc.
Suite 100, 1350 Center Drive
Dunwoody, Georgia 30338
(800) 728-2288

Contents

**Other Books by
William Campbell Douglass, M.D.:**

*AIDS: Why It's Much Worse Than They're Telling Us and
How To Protect Yourself and Your Loved Ones*

Dangerous Legal Drugs

*Eat Your Cholesterol: How to Live Off the Fat of the
Land and Feel Great*

Hydrogen Peroxide: Medical Miracle

Into the Light

The Milk Book

Introduction

The Problem

Bad medicine has been around for thousands of years. Patients have been poisoned, bled to death, dismembered, lied to, robbed, and purged since the first recording of history and, undoubtedly before that.

Of course, modern medicine is quite incredible in many ways. Ophthalmic surgery, orthopedics, and emergency medicine are but a few of the examples of superb modern medicine. But ironically the bad has kept pace with the good. Some of my critics would consider that an exaggeration, but when you consider the deplorable situation in cancer therapy, for instance, it seems obvious that we are going backward in many areas.

Of course many doctors are not consciously a part of the problem. Still, they have to survive in a system that rewards conflicts of interest, unnecessary treatments, and expensive, pointless diagnostic procedures, while practitioners of alternative, nontoxic therapies are persecuted and severely punished.

This report is meant to counteract the massive propaganda on your television where over half the commercials are for one drug or another, some bogus diet plan, or an anti-cholesterol product that will give you the very disease you are trying to avoid. I hope you'll find it useful.

Chapter 1

Sugar
The Truth about Hypoglycemia
and Diabetes

Dietary sugar is the root of more problems than the medical establishment has previously believed. In fact, it's *very* serious. When you consume heavy doses of sugar, your body reacts by producing abnormal insulin levels. This insulin, which is produced by your pancreas and controls your blood sugar level, rushes into your blood in response to that Rum Bavarian pie you just ate.

While the body needs the insulin to drive down the blood sugar, too much can have devastating effects on the body. High blood pressure, diabetes, and hypoglycemia are the most common repercussions of this hyperinsulinism. In fact, high concentrations of insulin are usually the cause of the distressful symptoms of "hypoglycemia" — not the low blood-sugar level, per se. These symptoms are well known and include weakness, dizziness, inability to think, "spaced out" feelings, jitteriness, heart palpitations, and irritability. In extreme cases, epileptic fits or maniacal behavior may occur. People have been admitted to mental institutions with a diagnosis of manic depression or schizophrenia because the diagnosis of hyperinsulinism was missed.

What this all boils down to is misdiagnosis by your doctor. *If you suffer classic "hypoglycemic" symptoms, but your doctor doesn't perform an insulin tolerance test along with the standard glucose tolerance test, the correct diagnosis may very well be missed.* You may go through life thinking you are crazy (or other people may think you are) when you are really suffering from hyperinsulinism.

Mistesting = Misdiagnosis

Let's look at the glucose tolerance test so you can see how doctors have been deluded into thinking that hypoglycemia is a rare condition sensationalized by health faddists.

After first taking a fasting blood sample ("fasting" in this case meaning no food intake for eight hours before the test), the patient is given a load of sugar in the form of a drink. The blood sugar is then measured every hour for five or six hours. His sugar level should be back to the fasting level (about 100) at the two-hour mark.

A normal glucose tolerance curve looks like this:

GRAPH A

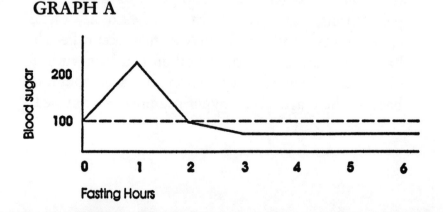

Confusion has reigned in this field because the results of the glucose tolerance test are often contradictory. If a patient has hypoglycemia — perhaps his blood sugar plummets to 42, as in graph B — then you would expect his symptoms to appear between the third and fifth hours, coincident with the low blood sugar. But he may experience weakness, shakiness, headache, etc., at hour two, as indicated on graph B, when his blood sugar is perfectly normal. So the doctor says: "You see? Your sugar was normal when you had your symptoms and *abnormal* when you felt OK, which proves that there is no such thing as hypoglycemia. It's all in your head."

GRAPH B

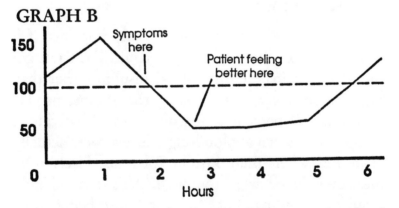

It's all in his head, all right. The excess insulin is affecting his brain. The pancreas excreted the insulin to counteract the sugar the doctor gave him. The insulin will have an immediate effect, while the sugar in the blood is still at a normal level — as shown in graph B. It's easy to prove this. Just hook the patient up to a brain-wave gadget called an electroencephalogram. His brain wave abnormalities will then be seen to coincide with his increased blood insulin levels.

In other words, because of mistesting the patient leaves the doctor's office, has a big meal including a gooey chocolate dessert, and starts feeling lousy. But now his problem is worse than before he saw the doctor. He not only feels bad physically, he also feels like a jerk because there is nothing wrong — the doctor said so. The next recourse is a psychiatrist, who will *really* mess up his head.

The Missing Link

The patient's case might be truly hopeless, if it weren't for the work of Dr. Joe Kraft. Dr. Kraft got the idea that maybe high blood insulin, rather than high blood sugar, was causing the symptoms. He found that 64 percent of so-called normal individuals (people with normal blood-sugar levels) were actually *abnormal* when their insulin tolerance levels were measured. They were too high. This was a highly significant finding, but, 16 years after being made public, most physicians still ignore it.

A doctor can be even further misled when the glucose tolerance test is perfectly normal, as in graph C. As shown, the insulin peak may come an hour or more after the blood sugar has returned to normal. If the doctor didn't do concurrent blood-insulin levels, he would conclude that your symptoms could not be related to sugar in your diet.

GRAPH C

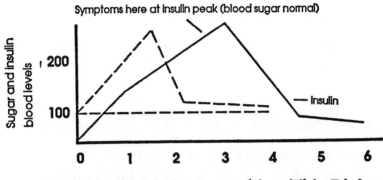

Symptoms here at insulin peak (blood sugar normal)

How Could They Miss Something This Big?

It's tragic to miss an early diagnosis of hypoglycemia, or worse, diabetes, because of failure to do an adequate lab test. It's also very ironic, when you consider how much unnecessary testing is done these days. Diabetes is one disease where early diagnosis really can make a difference. Failure to make an early diagnosis may lead to hypertension, hardening of the arteries, kidney disease, blindness, and premature death. Kraft proved that diet control, if instituted early enough, can bring insulin levels back to normal.

Insulin can cause no end of trouble — even the insulin the doctor prescribes for sugar control of a diabetic. We used to think that it didn't matter how much insulin a patient took on a daily basis, as long as the blood sugar was kept under control. This belief obviously assumed that *sugar* is the culprit responsible for ruining a patient's health, not *insulin*. Such thinking led to dietary nihilism: "You can eat anything you want as long as the insulin is keeping the blood sugar under control."

That was very bad dietary advice. But there's worse.

A 100-Year-Old "Quack" Cure for Diabetics?

For more than a hundred years doctors have been recommending the wrong foods for the control of blood sugar in diabetics. They thought they knew which foods a diabetic had to avoid to keep the blood sugar under control — ice cream, sugar, bread, etc. They were wrong. Doctors have been giving bad advice for 100 years based on *assumptions* that no one bothered to test on man or beast.

You probably won't believe this (and neither will your doctor), but Dr. J. A. Jenkins discovered, and Dr. Phyllis Crapo confirmed, that sugar and ice cream don't really affect the blood-sugar level dramatically. An Irish potato or a slice of whole wheat bread, however — things we thought were good for diabetics — can drive blood-sugar levels out of sight.

Incorrect dietary recommendations have led to the chasing of blood sugar levels with ever more insulin, which has in turn led to the many complications of diabetes. *This is important to you whether you have diabetes or not*, because this erroneous dietary advice is undoubtedly contributing to the rampancy of diabetes that we are seeing today. Correcting this single error could lead to a dramatic drop in the use of toxic antihypertensive drugs if doctors would follow through. But don't hold your breath.

Hyperinsulinism is by no means the only reason to avoid a heavy sugar intake. According to the sugar babies at the Food and Drug Administration, though, sugar is no big deal. They say sugar won't hurt you, aside from damage to your teeth. What they don't tell you is that sugar increases the white blood cell count (the body's reaction to a foreign invader), increases blood triglycerides (fat), lowers resistance to infection, decreases serum lysine (which contributes to osteoporosis) and, as you are now aware, increases serum insulin levels.

Researchers at the University of Connecticut found that 60 minutes following the ingestion of a sugar-laden fruit drink, preschool children showed a change for the worse in their performance and, demonstrated "inappropriate" behavior. That's a nice way of saying they became nasty little monsters. The one-hour reaction by the children corresponded to an elevated serum insulin level.

Action To Take:

(1)   Avoid foods that raise your blood sugar level (and so, secondarily, your blood insulin). The only practical way to do this is to get a glucometer (blood sugar tester) at your drug store, eat an Irish potato, for example, and test your blood sugar level every hour for five hours. It may be a lot of trouble, but it's more than worth it.

(2)   Ask your doctor to do a GITT — glucose-insulin tolerance test. If he expresses no interest in, or an antagonism for, the insulin test, tell him you want to see the results. This will shake him a little and force him to at least look at the report (doctors are wary of well-informed patients).

Chapter 2

Aspirin
The Bitter Pill That Kills

Aspirin is *in*. An aspirin promotion group called the Aspirin Foundation boasts that the chemical "probably has been taken, at one time or another, by almost every human being on earth."

Wishful thinking, no doubt, but pill-happy Americans scarf down *25 million aspirin tablets a day*. The British take it in a powder, the Italians take an effervescent, champagne-like mix, the French take it rectally, and the Thailanders put it in their morning and evening tea. Chemical companies produce *90 billion* aspirin tablets a year. If all those tablets were placed end to end they would stretch to the planet Infinity and back.

Did you ever think that you would see the day when Americans by the millions would be popping aspirin for their health? Do all these people really have an aspirin deficiency? Did God forget to put aspirin in our food? Will an aspirin a day keep the doctor away?

You'd probably say no to all of the above because it doesn't make any sense to take a chemical as if it were a vitamin. But it took the British to figure out how the aspirin industry and the AMA pulled off such a scam.

The Real Hero: Magnesium

The much-promoted Physician's Health Study proving that taking aspirin regularly will prevent heart attacks didn't use just aspirin but aspirin *plus magnesium* in the form of Bufferin.

Research done years ago proved that magnesium protects the heart. It dilates blood vessels, aids in absorption of potassium into cells (which will prevent heartbeat irregularities), acts as an anticoagulant (blood thinner) and keeps the blood cells from sticking together (thrombosis). Autopsy of the heart muscle following death by heart attack almost always reveals that the heart muscle is deficient in magnesium.

I have been taking a magnesium supplement (K-Mag from Vitaline — there are other good ones) for 10 years and I have hundreds of patients on magnesium. We just don't see heart attacks in patients who stick with it.

So the doctors (and their patients) have been conned again by the group that has been leading them around by the nose for 75 years — the pharmaceutical industry. A British study using *only* aspirin revealed that aspirin had *absolutely nothing* to do with lowering the incidence of heart attacks.

Robbing Peter to Pay Paul?

The American study was so flawed that you can't help but wonder if the aspirin industry financed it. The subjects were white, male, mostly non- smoking doctors who were not monitored, and who reported their condition by letter — post office research. The study used an extremely healthy group with only *one-eighth* the death rate of the general population.

Even with such a healthy group, the study results had some ominous overtones. That's the part the aspirin companies don't want you to know about. Though heart attacks were relatively rare, strokes and sudden death from other causes were more common among the aspirin group than with the placebo group.

This information is very significant. The claim for reduction in heart attacks among the aspirin group was 47 percent. But the small print (*very* small print) in the report said that when death from all causes was considered, there was *no difference* in the mortality rates of the two groups. Thus, *death from other causes among the aspirin group increased substantially — an amount equal to 47 percent of all heart attacks in the non-aspirin group.*

Did you know that every time you take aspirin you bleed a little into your gut? A microscope will show that the bowel movement of someone on daily aspirin has blood in it every time. If it's happening in your intestinal tract, how do you know it's not happening in your brain? How many strokes are precipitated by chronic aspirin intake? How many fatal hemorrhages of the brain, spleen, liver, intestine, or lung occur after an automobile accident because the blood has been thinned with aspirin? Nobody knows and nobody is checking.

Prevention That Works

There are many natural ways to protect yourself from heart attack without enriching the Bayer Company:

- *Magnesium*, as mentioned above, is absolutely essential for a healthy heart and should be given credit for the beneficial results obtained in the aspirin study.
- *Salmon oil* contains a strong platelet anti-sticking agent called eicosapentaenoic acid (EPA).
- *Garlic* blocks the clotting mechanism.
- *Niacin* is a well known anti-atherosclerotic agent.
- *Vitamin C* is an important factor in prostaglandin production.
- *Vitamin E* is also important in the production of prostaglandins.
- *Bromelin* reduces platelet stickiness.
- *Zinc* is a necessary catalyst, along with the enzyme d-6-d, in certain fatty acid metabolic

processes essential to the health of your coronary arteries.

- *Vitamin B-6* (pyridoxine) converts the highly atherogenic homocysteine to cystathionine. This prevents meat protein from damaging your arteries. Also stops platelet aggregation.
- *Folic Acid* neutralizes the enzyme XO in homogenized pasteurized milk. XO hardens your arteries.
- *Carnitine* and *Taurine,* two of the amino acids considered nonessential by most nutritionists, are absolutely essential for a healthy heart.

There are other nutrients for a healthy heart, but you get the picture. So who needs aspirin?

The Cancer Connection

A few years ago I was in Nashville, Tennessee attending a medical conference with a colleague. While at dinner he developed severe chest pain, was rushed to the university hospital, and was found to have suffered a heart attack. He went very quickly to bypass surgery and survived it with no complications.

I was visiting him one day following the surgery when a nurse came in to give him his aspirin tablet. She stood there and watched him take it with a glass of water. It was almost a ritual. Such is the reverence felt for this drug.

But in addition to the reports showing aspirin has no preventive effect on heart attacks, new reports show that aspirin may cause cancer. And what's more, a study of California researchers reported in the British Medical Journal that older men and women who take aspirin every day almost double their chances of developing so-called ischemic heart disease. Ischemic heart disease accounts for a wide range of illnesses involving blockage of the arteries carrying blood to the heart.

Aspirin-users were also more likely to develop kidney and colon cancer, the study found.

Lawrence Garfinkel, Vice President for Epidemiology at the American Cancer Society said, "It would give one pause about using aspirin routinely to prevent an initial heart attack. This is going to be very confusing to the public. "The new study concluded: "Our study would not recommend that these people routinely consume aspirin."

There are a few other reasons why you shouldn't take aspirin: indigestion, bleeding ulcers with possible hemorrhage and death from exsanguination (internal bleeding) and hemorrhagic stroke.

I'm Vain About My Brain

Leo Dropperman started taking aspirin to prevent a second heart attack, as advised by his doctor and the

TV commercials. But when he read that daily doses could increase his chances of getting a hemorrhagic stroke, he quit. "I'd much rather have a heart attack than a stroke," said the Tennessee psychologist. "I'm very vain about my brain."

Of course, it may be even worse than that. The British report mentioned earlier found no beneficial effect on heart attack frequency from taking aspirin, but the California study goes even further in suggesting that daily aspirin use may actually *increase* the odds of having a heart attack, as well as give you kidney and colon cancer.

On hearing that news, drug companies quickly folded their medicine tents and split. Their commercials connecting aspirin with beneficial effects on heart disease were scrapped. Sterling Drug (Eastman Kodak) pulled its commercial depicting the Bayer aspirin logo over a pulsating heart monitor and substituted the old logo: "the wonder drug doctors themselves take more often for pain." Bristol-Myers dragged out Angela Lansbury to say: "A cup of tea and a couple of Bufferin allow me to do the things I want to do." Sterling Drugs even went so far as to introduce a Bayer calendar pack to remind people to take their aspirin.

Consumers are beginning to question all these contradictory studies. They don't know who to believe anymore. So, when it comes to advice on drugs, who *can* you trust? The FDA? Well, in

December, 1984 the FDA recommended allowing drug companies to promote the use of aspirin to reduce the chances of a second heart attack.

Can you trust the medical journals? In January, 1988, the *New England Journal of Medicine* reported that an aspirin every other day reduced the risk of heart attacks. (Is it coincidental that the drug companies have been able to get their slimy fingers into the *New England Journal of Medicine* with multi-million-dollar advertising contracts?)

Can you trust the medical advice given by actors on TV commercials? Forget I asked.

Can you trust the hospitals and their doctors? Remember the episode my colleague had in the hospital with the nurse force-feeding him aspirin?

After the aspirin-popping media blitz, aspirin sales temporarily increased and then resumed the old downward trend. The news leaked out that an aspirin a day would keep good health away. One disgusted advertising drummer said plaintively: "About the only preventive thing people do in this country is brush their teeth with fluoride."

I guess you can't trust the advertising agencies either.

Chapter 3

Dangerous Dentistry
Fillings That Can Make You Ill

I warned about the dangers of silver amalgam fillings over four years ago. Now that 60 Minutes has come out with an exposé on these mercury-containing restoratives, we are witnessing the slow retreat of the American Dental Association from their unqualified support of silver/mercury fillings.

You see, "silver" isn't silver when you are talking dentistry. It is lead, tin, mercury and a little silver. I've been recommending "gold" in place of "silver," but now I have to put gold in quotes, too, because "gold" isn't gold. Much to my chagrin, I've found out that nickel and beryllium, both toxic, are often mixed with the gold. Some of the material billed as gold contains as little as two percent of the precious metal. (But you and the dentist pay for it as if it were pure gold.)

The ADA has been stonewalling the issue of mercury amalgam toxicity for years. In fact, until seven years ago, the ADA said *no vapor at all* was released from these fillings. But when the public got wind of the fact that mercury/silver fillings can damage their health, the ADA met the issue head on. It denied that there was any danger and started persecuting (and prosecuting) dentists who strayed from the party line.

In dentistry, there has been a complete breakdown in constitutional rights. Dentists who have spoken out have been ruined by having their licenses revoked, without benefit of a jury trial or any other pretense of protecting their rights. Dr. Murray Vimy, a professor at the University of Calgary Medical School who is himself a dentist, said: "The effect has been that, in the United States, the constitutional rights of dentists and the rights of patients have been taken away. They no longer have freedom of choice and they no longer have freedom of expression."

It's All About Power

You see, despite the public's perception, scientists are generally very narrow-minded and bigoted, and dentists are no exception. This generalization applies especially to those in a position of power in a scientific organization. They are more interested in power and control than they are science. If they were more interested in science than power, they would stick to science and not seek power — an axiomatic statement if there ever was one. So, naturally, dentists will ferociously resist a new idea, especially if the new idea implies that they have been doing something wrong for a hundred years. They are human, after all, and who wants to look stupid?

A typical defense of mercury fillings is the letter that Drs. Golden and Golden sent to their patients:

> Considering the millions of patients who have been treated over that period (of 150 years) and the billions of fillings that have been placed, the fact that there has not been a worldwide epidemic of mercury-related diseases with reports of widespread poisoning is reassurance enough that there is no danger to health from dental amalgam in teeth....

Keeping in mind that the Goldens are dentists, not toxicologists or clinical physicians, let's look at what the textbook, *Goodman and Gilman's The Pharmacological Basis of Therapeutics*, the bible of pharmacology, has to say about mercury poisoning. According to its authors, mercury poisoning epidemics often go misdiagnosed for years because of, in their words, "the vagueness of early clinical signs" and the medical profession's "unfamiliarity with the disease."

This being the case, are dentists qualified to make a statement that "there is no danger to health from dental amalgam in teeth"?

As Dr. Alfred Zamm said on "60 Minutes," "Doctors very rarely make a diagnosis of mercury poisoning because of the difficulties of it. It [has] different faces. One [patient] has headaches, one has tiredness, one has this, one has that. It's a very difficult diagnosis to make, especially when it's micro-mercurialism, very small amounts." Dr. Zamm is an allergist and dermatologist and has reported *hundreds of cases* of patients who have recovered from a variety of diseases after having their fillings removed.

The Goldens go on to say in their letter:

It is in dentists' financial interest to do work that is medically necessary. [That's not necessarily so, either] But to endorse such a policy [mercury fillings] with no acceptable scientific evidence to support it, would be not only unethical, but also dangerous to the public health and to dentists' professional reputation.

They are precisely right. It *is* unethical because there is "no acceptable scientific evidence to support it;" it *is* dangerous to the public health and it is *most definitely* dangerous to dentists' professional reputation.

There's very strong evidence that mercury in dental fillings can cause a broad spectrum of symptoms and diseases. Everything from depression to arthritis may be involved in a particular case; it's extremely variable. Mercury poisoning has been implicated in Alzheimer's disease, colitis, kidney disease, birth defects, brain damage, and symptoms of multiple sclerosis. *And the more you brush your mercury fillings the worse the toxicity becomes.* (Believe it or not, one of the best things you can do for your teeth is to throw away your toothbrush — it doesn't prevent tooth decay, it wears off your enamel and it stirs up your mercury. Use a water pik-type instrument with three percent hydrogen peroxide to clean your teeth.)

Who Says There's No Evidence?

Faye Dores had crippling arthritis, colitis, fatigue and memory loss. At age 35, she was told that she would soon be confined to a wheelchair for life. Faye had her dentist check her mouth for mercury vapor. The level was so astronomical that, if she had been a building, the Environmental Protection Agency would have had to condemn her and tear her down. She had her mercury fillings removed. In three weeks, she threw away her cane; her tremors stopped and the swelling went out of her joints. She states that she is 95 percent cured.

Nancy Yost of San Jose, California, was told by her doctors that she had multiple sclerosis. The diagnosis was confirmed by tests and she was declared "incurable." She had worked in the dental industry and so knew about mercury toxicity. Her doctors had told her to "get real" and not to expect too much out of life. In other words, give up.

As a last resort, she had her five mercury fillings removed. She left the dentist's office using a cane and leaning heavily on the arm of a friend. The next day she went to her doctor and threw her cane at him. The next night she went dancing. She has some lingering effects but was basically cured by the removal of the "silver" fillings.

Somebody Created a Monster

How could this disastrous situation have developed? Doesn't the Food and Drug Administration protect us from arrogant and irresponsible scientists as well as contaminated food? Unfortunately, at least in the case of dentistry, the answer is *no*. The FDA's dental division is stacked with people from the American Dental Association and they tell the FDA what to do where dental regulation is concerned. There is virtually no medical input or basic science, such as toxicology — which is what we are talking about here — represented on the FDA's dental board. So your health is in the hands of a bunch of political dentists who know *nothing* about mercury toxicity.

Perhaps this explains why *100 million* mercury fillings were put in American mouths last year and yet this amalgam has never been tested by the FDA for safety — it got automatic approval. Perhaps this explains why the FDA refused to be interviewed by

"60 Minutes" concerning the mercury amalgam issue. They issued a statement which said: "The FDA remains confident in the value of amalgams in dental care." Notice that the word *mercury* was left out of the statement. Maybe it was an oversight.

It would be a little harsh to say that dentists don't know what they are doing. But they are not aware of the content of the metals they use to repair your fillings. Whether the material is so-called gold or so-called silver, the dentist really doesn't know what combination of metals he is putting in your mouth.

Your dentist has been duped by the dental laboratories that make the metal mixtures. The content of the gold in the gold alloys may vary from 80 percent down to two percent. You can rest assured that the metals added are cheaper than gold but the dentist is charged the gold price. There are 400 alloys billed as gold and your dentist hasn't the slightest idea what he is packing into your teeth.

There are 10,000 laboratories in the U.S. making every conceivable combination of metal filling in this *two billion dollar* business. John Williams, president of Gold Refining Company, told the *Wall Street Journal*: "The dentists are confused. They don't understand what they are getting. Essentially, it's our fault. We created a flock of alloys." He could have said, "we created a monster."

The insurance companies aren't happy, either. An official of Aetna Life said, "We don't know what we are paying for because the dentists don't know what they use."

Grudgingly, the ADA is shimmying back from the end of the dental amalgam limb. Delegates of the American Dental Association announced that they will consider whether to endorse a plan to identify what is actually in the stuff the dentist is putting in your teeth. That's not exactly an admission of error or ignorance, but it's a start. Or is it? While making this new show of scientific curiosity (What have we actually been using to fill teeth these last 100 years?), the ADA continues to urge state dental associations to fight any legislation that would require dentists to explain to patients the risks of amalgam fillings.

What Mercury Does

We'll come back to the stiff-necks of the ADA in a moment. But first let's take a closer look at mercury.

Mercury is universally acknowledged to be an extremely poisonous element. Data from occupational exposure shows that the toxic effects of mercury vapor are well known. The wisdom of using a known toxin as a dental restorative material in so-called silver amalgams should be questioned on this basis alone.

Mercury is more poisonous than lead, cadmium, or arsenic. Yet, no dentist would dream of packing your teeth with lead or arsenic. Inhaled mercury vapor is at least a hundred times more toxic than swallowed mercury. Mercury vapor is what comes off your teeth from the fillings when you chew your food. This occurs multiple times a day every time you eat or grind your teeth together. Also, a battery-like effect, resulting from two metal fillings touching each other, can cause a continuous release of mercury vapor into your mouth.

The body has no mechanism for releasing this toxic metal so it is stored in your bones, your kidneys and your brain. No wonder some people can't remember their own zip code.

Mercury-vapor levels in the mouth remain *for an hour or longer.* An individual with mercury amalgam fillings having three meals and three snacks a day, will extrapolate to *over the Occupational, Safety and Health Act's toxic limit for a 40-hour work week and over the EPA's maximum allowable concentration for mercury vapor.*

In other words, his mouth is a toxic waste dump.

When mercury vapor is inhaled, it reaches the brain almost instantaneously. Autopsy studies have shown a positive correlation between the amounts of mercury found in the brain and the number of amalgams found in the mouth. A similar correlation has been found with the pituitary gland, the master gland in your head that controls about everything else, including your thyroid and adrenal glands.

Problem? What Problem?

Don't let your dentist reassure you with a blood-level test for mercury. The test is not reliable and tells you nothing about the amount of mercury that your body has stored over the years. Claiming you have no mercury problem on the basis of a blood-level test is like claiming you have no cockroaches in your house because you can't see any — maybe you're right, and maybe not.

Dr. Heber Simmons, consumer adviser for the American Dental Association, was asked by Morley Safer, "You concede that there is a constant release of mercury vapor [from amalgam fillings]?"

> Oh, we don't dispute that at all. [Very convenient. Remember, the ADA's position till seven years ago was to totally deny any vapor release.] But the amount that is being released when you chew is such a small amount that it is not going to cause a problem.

When asked to explain the remarkable recoveries we described earlier, Simmons retorted that the cases were anecdotal and clinically insignificant.

There is nothing anecdotal about the sheep studies done at the University of Calgary. Six mature sheep were given mercury amalgam fillings identical to what your dentist uses. *All six of the sheep lost half their kidney function within 30 days of receiving the fillings.* The same results were obtained with monkeys. Further, the researchers noted that the monkeys' immune systems were severely injured.

Ironically, Dr. Simmons of the ADA is a pediatric dentist, meaning he gets the mercury into his patients early in life, almost guaranteeing health problems later. He thinks the mercury controversy is just a cruel hoax.

Maybe Simmons should have *his* teeth examined.

Action to Take:

Buy a cheap dental mirror at the drug store and check your teeth in good light. If you have grayish-looking fillings, they are probably silver amalgam. It is not always easy for a layman to tell. If you are not sure, call the International Academy of Oral Medicine and Toxicology in Colorado Springs, Colorado, at (719) 599-8883. They can direct you to a dentist in your area who is experienced with the mercury toxicity problem.

Chapter 4

Fluoridation
Don't Drink That Water

Fluoridation of public water supplies is certainly one of the sacred cows of this century. Every expert on the subject from the American Dental Association to the local dentist says fluoride is essential for arresting or preventing tooth decay. Its position as the wonder drug of dental science is virtually sacrosanct. Yet the facts of the matter, repressed by those with vested interests in the fluoride industry, strongly contradict common wisdom on the subject.

Because fluoride is linked to an increase in cardiovascular disease and cancer, an increase in dental and gum pathology, and has been proven to have no effect on tooth decay, Sweden, Holland, and Germany have discontinued fluoridation of their water supplies. In fact, because of serious health concerns, fluoridation has been terminated or never implemented in almost every country in continental Europe. Yet American dentists continue to tell their patients that fluoridation of water is beyond scientific debate.

Dentists claim that fluoridation reduces tooth decay by 50 percent and is absolutely safe. Absolutely safe? According to internal documents obtained from the Environmental Protection Agency (EPA), fluoride may soon be classified as a *carcinogen*.

John H. Sullivan, deputy executive director of the American Water Works Association, remarked:

> If fluoride turns out to be a carcinogen, it will be the environmental story of the century. And if our members have to start removing fluoride from drinking water, their job will be mind-boggling.

The propaganda by the ADA for fluoridation has been so pervasive that the average American thinks of fluoride as an essential nutrient. Until March 16, 1979, the Food and Drug Administration (FDA), also taken in by the dentists and the fluoridation lobby, actually had fluoride listed as an essential or possibly essential nutrient. Yet countless studies have shown this to be untrue.

One such study examined the Australian aborigines, whose diet is high in refined sugar. They have a very high incidence of cavities, in spite of the fact that their water is naturally fluoridated. So the cause of dental (and gum) problems is not a lack of fluoride in water and toothpaste (now they are even fluoridating milk), but our high sugar diets. The study merely confirms what most of us have known for quite some time.

In New Zealand, the only city that is not fluoridated is Christchurch. Yet, there is no *significant difference* in the average amount of tooth decay found in Christchurch compared with the fluoridated cities of New Zealand. In fact, by 1966, when fluoridation was well entrenched in New Zealand, tooth decay was an already rapidly disappearing problem.

John Yiamouyiannis, one of the pioneers in the anti-fluoridation movement, obtained information through the Freedom of Information Act that proved there was no significant difference in the decay rate of children's teeth in fluoridated and unfluoridated cities in the United States. A study in Missouri showed the same result: *No difference* in average levels of tooth decay between fluoridated and unfluoridated cities.

In Canada the studies are even more telling. In the province of British Columbia, which is only 11 percent fluoridated, there is *less* tooth decay than in other provinces that are 40-70 percent fluoridated.

The original studies of fluoridation, which were used to sell the people of the world (especially the U.S., Australia, and New Zealand) on fluoridation, were based on chicanery and deceit. In one English study the control group was chosen 19 years *after* the fluoridation experiment was started. For controls, they chose an urban area known for its high rate of tooth decay, whereas the experimental group was chosen from a rural area known for a low rate of tooth decay. After 19 years, the fluoride experimental group had fewer cavities just as they had two decades previously without fluoridation. That's called creative science.

The most blatant example of cheating and fudging was uncovered in a trial in Hastings, New Zealand. There it was found that a claimed decline in tooth decay resulted from instructions to dental therapists *to find and fill fewer cavities*. Naturally, this was never mentioned in published reports of the trial and was only brought to light when a whistle-blower requested the information under the New Zealand Official Information Act.

There are over 20 studies showing that tooth decay has been declining just as rapidly in unfluoridated cities as in fluoridated cities around the world. The fluoride lobby has withheld this vital information, not only from you, but also from the dental profession. Such malfeasance has led well-meaning dentists to continue to promote a toxic waste product that has damaged the health of tens of millions of people all over the world.

Although the use of topical fluoride (that applied directly to the teeth) is questionable (and entirely unnecessary with a low-sugar diet), good research has proven that taking fluoride internally has no positive health benefits for your teeth, but can have devastating effects on your general health (more on that later).

Government Experts See No Evil

After 40 years of constant and costly clamoring, the anti-fluoride forces have made a major breakthrough. The doubts about the safety and the efficacy of fluoridated water have become so overwhelming that the Surgeon General was forced to convene a world-class group of experts to review the literature on the health effects of fluoride in drinking water. The following interesting quotes are from these experts who are supposed to know about the effects of fluoride on human health:

"If you are talking about potential toxicity, we have no idea whether it is 18 or puberty. We have no idea." (Michael Kleerekoper, M.D., Henry Ford Hospital, Detroit, Michigan.)

"I just don't know where the truth is. That is what I don't know." (J.R. Shapiro, M.D., Clinical Center, National Institutes of Health, Washington, D.C.)

"I realize we have few facts and many unknowns...." (Stanley Wallach, M.D., V.A. Medical Center, Albany, New York.)

The above report, with its interesting comments, *was suppressed for over five years* until Martha Bevis of Houston, with the aid of her congressman, obtained a copy of it.

So 40 years after they began dumping fluoride into our water, and after tens of thousands of people have protested and spent millions of dollars trying to stop the madness, it comes out in this suppressed report that no one knew, and still no one knows, what is being done to people with the fluoridation of water. (Actually, they know *a lot* and the experts are running for cover.)

Even before these startling admissions, a 1979 study by the Centers for Disease Control revealed that more than half of water companies were adding either too much or too little fluoride, according to the recommended standards.

Doctors discussed crippling endemic bone fluorosis at this secret meeting. They admitted they had no idea what level of fluoride would cause this terrible condition, but it was obvious that many water supplies had a high enough concentration to induce the disease. It was concluded that this diagnosis was not being made more often simply because doctors weren't aware of it.

Commenting on a condition called osteosclerosis, found almost exclusively in overfluoridated people, the doctors admitted they did not know what fluoride was doing to the bones or the rest of the body. They simply called it a potential adverse effect.

Dr. Shapiro added: "Let's just say that because we really don't have the information ... osteosclerosis occurs and we really don't know whether it is potentially adverse or not. We don't have the data."

Millions of children in the United States have had their teeth disfigured from fluoride by a condition called fluorosis. Dr. Robert Marcus reported at the meeting:

> I think it is fairly close to unanimous that we agree that dental fluorosis, in fact, has medical ramifications. Not knowing where bone disease begins at any age, what you are saying is that if there is something going on in the teeth, then the likelihood is that there is something going on in the bones. You don't know that it is there; you don't know that it is *not* there.

The astounding conclusion of the group, a conclusion that is remarkably similar to what many Americans have been saying for 40 years, is that the fluoride levels of possible health significance are quite low. Put another way: it doesn't take much fluoride to adversely affect your health. Dr. Shapiro pointed out there is a town in Texas where children with severe fluorosis were drinking water with a fluoride level of only 1.2 parts per million well within the safe range.

The panel continued to fumble around the issue of what is safe and what is not safe. It was suggested that children should take a level of fluoride of two parts per million or less, and not four parts per million as has been recommended safe for adults. This would mean that you would have to have a water tap in your kitchen marked children and another one marked adults.

Dr. Kleerekoper continued to throw a wet blanket over the proceeding by pointing out: "From all the available data, we can't state that there is no apparent adverse health effect of a water fluoride level of two parts per million or below."

Dr. Wallach was even more specific: "You would have to have rocks in your head, in my opinion, to allow your children much more than two parts per million."

Then the committee took up the issue of the cutoff age for the lower dose of two parts per million. Referring to the age at which fluoride usage becomes toxic, Dr. Marcus stated, *"I would make it very, very clear that we know nothing about this issue."*

Dr. Beth Dawson Hughes said, "I am not sure a ten-year-old is going to have no harm from four parts per million. I am not sure what it is going to do to their bone turnover rate and to the concerns that have been expressed."

Then a vote was taken (remember, in bureaucratic medicine you don't do scientific studies, you vote), and Dr. Wallach said, "I know I mentioned every age under the sun. I guess I'll settle with a recommendation for age 18 [for recommended low fluoride dose]." On a vote of five to four, the committee split that recommendation down the middle and settled for the age of nine.

Then the committee performed its most astounding (and typically political) maneuver. After their agonizing admission of ignorance ("we have no idea," "we just don't have the data," "we just don't know," etc.), *they completely eviscerated their own recommendations and conclusions and vouched absolutely, unequivocally that fluoride levels of four parts per million were perfectly safe!*

With the utter fecklessness revealed by this study, it is no wonder the national water fluoridation program is showing signs of decay. Topical application of a little flimflam just won't sell any more. Forty percent of U.S. water supplies remain unfluoridated in spite of continual, taxpayer-financed, pro-fluoridation propaganda. The government is now giving the brush-off to proponents of fluoridation, promising them no further funding.

In spite of the American Dental Association's relentless drive for near universal fluoridation by the year 2000, the tide has turned and the American people are rejecting fluoride. The we-just-don't-know-but-you-should-use-it-in-large-doses-anyway recommendation of the Surgeon General's committee may be good politics but it can hardly be called science.

Fluoride and America's Children

Fluoridation proponents prefer to talk about concentration, i.e., parts per million, rather than dosage, which is really all that matters — how much fluoride is the person actually getting? Breast milk contains only about 0.01 parts per million fluoride, depending on the quantity of fluoride ingested by the mother. Infants who are bottle-fed on powdered formula reconstituted with fluoridated water ingest *100 times* the dose of fluoride ingested by breast-fed babies. The most obvious impact of this enormous unnatural fluoride dose is the development of disfigured teeth, fluorosis, in a majority of the babies exposed. The less obvious impact will be the development of bone cancer, mouth cancer, arthritis, neurological disease, or cardiovascular disease later in life.

After the bottle stage, the child does not escape hyperfluoridation. Dentists educate the parents on the importance of training their children to brush their teeth "after every meal." Few do it, of course, because most people just aren't that compulsive. That's fortunate for the children, because even brushing once a day results in the ingestion of massive amounts of fluoride from swallowing the super sweet toothpaste — they love it.

Another major problem affecting two and a half million Americans is fluoride allergy. Allergic reactions to fluoride may include: nausea, vomiting and abdominal pain, skin rash, (even from bathing in fluoridated water), mouth sores (including those from fluoridated toothpaste), headaches, arthritic pains, dryness of the throat, excessive water consumption (polyuria), chronic fatigue, depression, nervousness, and respiratory difficulties.

Action to Take

(1) Don't drink water from the tap unless you have a tested well of your own.
(2) Buy bottled water of known purity. Remember that the bottling company doesn't have to tell you on the label about the fluoride content of their water but they are required to keep the information on file for your inquiry.
(3) Get a good reverse osmosis filter that will remove fluoride, radon, and chlorine (that's another story).
(4) Ask your congressman where he stands on the fluoridation issue and tell him that you want him to take a stand against fluoride poisoning of the water supply.

The Moral and Constitutional Issue

James J. Kilpatrick, in his syndicated column, has made some telling remarks about the morality of the fluoridation issue:

The deeper issue is now, and always has been, the issue of personal freedom. Whatever may be said for fluoridation as a matter of public health, the program is a patent invasion of private rights specifically, the right of each individual to control the medicine he takes.

The power of the state is invoked to make us ingest what most dentists say is good for us. Doctor knows best. So shut up.

The law forbids us from taking cocaine. Fluoridation compels us to take fluoride. The one is seen as an evil; the other is seen as good. But it is one thing to forbid and quite another thing to compel. This is the issue that matters.

Thirty years ago many of us were bashed, trashed and called lunatics for opposing fluoridation. I wish Kilpatrick had written this fine editorial in 1960 instead of 1990. But better late than never.

Chapter 5

Exercise
Stop Sweating and Add Years
to Your Life

Everyone knows exercise will make you healthy, cause you to lose weight, prevent heart attacks, help your sex life, and increase your life span. Everyone also knew the world was flat.

I have a friend who seems to be allergic to exercise. He says he gets most of his aerobics by serving as a pallbearer for his hyperactive friends. Perhaps a little hyperbole there, but it deserves thought; I've had many a friend drop dead on the tennis court.

Exercise may increase your *fitness* without improving your health. Pumping iron may blow up your muscles, but there is no evidence that I'm aware of that it improves basic physiology. To me, a trip to the weight room is like a trip to hell. And women just aren't designed for some of those exercises, especially those involving stress on the shoulder girdle. If you insist on doing these mindless exercises, ladies, watch out for your shoulders.

After bypass surgery, the surgeon places the patient on a very organized and stringent exercise program. This increases fitness and endurance, giving the patient the illusion of vast improvement from the surgery. Within two years, half of these patients will have their dreams shattered by another heart attack.

I took care of a retired electrician when I was in medical school. All his life, he never picked up anything heavier than a screwdriver and he was proud of it. I was a senior when we buried him — at age 93. My maternal grandmother weighed 250 pounds most of her life. She got her exercise peeling potatoes and maintaining a country home in rural Georgia. She never heard of aerobics. She died at 85.

American business is into jogging, squashing, pumping iron, and handballing. But one business cynic remarked: Our executives look marvelous and they say they feel great. Of course, they don't do much because they're tired from all that running. Maybe that's one reason American business, once the pride of the civilized world, is fading fast. Should we give running shoes to the Japanese? Get 'em out of the office and into the street? Nothing else has worked.

Jogging doesn't even appear to be safe for *professional athletes.* New York Yankee catcher Elston Howard, body builder Charles Atlas, Paavo Nurmi, the Flying Finn, Olympian John Kelly and the greatest jogger of them all, Jim Fixx, all died of heart attacks while jogging, and that's just a partial list. An amazing number of professional athletes die young and the reason may be because of their abnormal and excessive exertion and not in spite of it. In fact, athletes frequently have abnormal electrocardiogram manifesting changes that would be accepted as evidence of heart disease in non-athletes.

Dr. Paul Thompson, *et al*, investigated the circumstances of death in 18 people who died during, or immediately after, jogging. Fourteen of the 18 individuals had exercised regularly for one or more years. Most of these were noncompetitive runners just doing their ordinary thing. But among marathon runners, those supposed to be protected from heart disease because of their superior fitness, the story is even worse: Severe coronary artery disease is the most common cause of death among marathoners!

Stress Test Dangers

What about that stress test used by your doctor to prescribe the amount of exercise you should have? It is not only useless but often harmful. The implication is that the doctor, because of his vast and intimate knowledge of your body, especially when armed with your cardiac stress test results, can order the amount and type of exercise that is right for your needs. This is a myth. Much of what you hear about stress testing is misinformation.

Stress testing was designed to (1) confirm the presence or absence of heart disease, and (2) establish a safe level of exercise for the patient. It does neither, and may produce misinformation, often with disastrous consequences. A study from the National Institutes of Health found that among 39 subjects who had no symptoms of heart disease but had clearly abnormal stress tests, only 36 percent had significant heart disease on more definitive testing, including dye x-ray examination of the arteries of the heart.

The stress test isn't even reproducible. Investigators were dismayed to find that repeating the stress test in the same individual would produce a different result about 50 percent of the time! Dr. Henry Solomon has remarked:

> On the basis of your medical history alone, an accurate enough estimate of the likelihood that you have coronary disease can be made. A stress test does not offer significant additional information. It may offer only additional confusion, and is therefore quite unnecessary.

But the situation with stress testing is even more dismaying than that. A certain number of people who prove to have perfectly normal hearts experience sudden death during treadmill stress testing. These disasters are probably caused by spasm of the coronary arteries. If your doctor suggests tread mill stress testing, tell him you have a bad knee.

There are many studies that "prove" a vigorous lifestyle increases longevity. But these studies were found to be seriously flawed. On closer examination, it was discovered that more vigorous men chose more physically challenging occupations to begin with. Sedentary, fat men chose sedentary jobs. So the healthier men didn't live longer because of their more physical occupations but because they were more healthy to begin with.

Some studies even show an inverse relationship between the physical demands of an occupation and longevity. An analysis of Indian railway workers in 1967 contributed to dispelling the exercise myth. The researchers reported "an unexpected and extraordinary finding in our data that mortality in the sedentary occupation of clerks is lower than the physically active occupation of fitters.... This is contrary to the current conceptions of the protective role of exercise."

A Scandinavian study in 1976 comparing several levels of activity of Finnish men found that total mortality was *highest* for men doing the most vigorous physical activity.

A 1975 report from Sweden covered 315 heart attack patients who were randomly assigned either to an exercise training program or to no program. There was no evident influence of exercise on either the death rate or the rate of recurrent heart attacks.

Reflecting on the above studies, Dr. Solomon, an experienced cardiologist and author, said:

The whole scientific community, cardiologists like myself especially, would like to promise that exercise removes the fatty obstructions from artery walls, reduces the pressure of blood against them, and keeps the juices flowing. But we can't. There simply is no evidence to support those hopes. As far as prevention of atherosclerosis or protection from its consequences is concerned, exercise will get you nowhere.

For women the addiction to running is far more serious than with men. Women who run miles every day lose significant amounts of calcium and are thus prone to early osteoporosis. The thin ones, and most female runners are thin, are more prone to get osteoporosis in the first place. The menstrual cycle is severely disturbed by compulsive running and at least 10 percent of women engaging in this quest for eternal youth have menstrual problems. Women who train the most and weigh the least tend to have few or no menstrual cycles. This adds even further to the risk of osteoporosis.

Are cardiac surgeons killing some of their patients with these extreme exercise programs following surgery? Is there any rationale behind overloading an already damaged heart? Dr. Solomon: "Even people with imminently fatal heart disease can play sports, exercise and run. They have no symptoms and may be capable of outstanding physical performance with hearts that will kill them."

If you want to exercise, *walk*. It's by far the safest and most pleasant way to exercise your body. The patients I've had who lived the longest were walkers. Some of them walked one to five miles a day — at a leisurely pace. What's the hurry?

Here's the bad news:

(1) Running will improve your "fitness" but not your heart.

(2) Stress testing is useless and dangerous to your health.

(3) There is no reliable evidence that exercise will prolong your life.

(4) Studs (of both sexes) who blow up their muscles through exercise do not necessarily live longer and may die sooner.

(5) Women are especially at risk from excessive exercise.

(6) Cardiac catastrophe is the overwhelming danger of vigorous exercise.

(7) Severe coronary atherosclerosis is the most common cause of death in marathon runners.

(8) Regular exercise does not prevent the development of coronary atherosclerosis.

(9) People don't die in spite of exercise. They die because of it.

(10) The statistics show overwhelmingly that sudden death is most likely to occur after strenuous exertion.

(11) Big-muscled, outdoors types do not live longer or have fewer heart attacks than sedentary office workers.

(12) The annual death rate for joggers is seven times that of people engaging in less strenuous exercise.

Here's the good news:

(1) You don't have to torture yourself anymore. Take up table tennis, croquet, or volleyball — lighten up.

(2) This report may have saved your life: The first marathoner was Pheidippides. He ran the 26 miles and 385 yards from Marathon to Athens to announce the victory over Persia at the Battle of Marathon. He announced the victory and promptly dropped dead.

So couch potatoes arise! No, on second thought, don't arise. Just stop smoking, eat fresh, undercooked food, limit your sugar intake, don't drink homogenized milk or chlorinated/ fluoridated water, and you'll be okay.

Chapter 6

Unnecessary Testing
Is Your Doctor Getting a Piece
of the Action?

Physicians in every community in the United States are supplementing their shrinking incomes with profits from interests in laboratories, X-ray centers and other medical facilities to which they refer their patients. This obvious conflict of interest is legal in most states, although the American Medical Association gives lip service to opposing it.

These kickbacks or scams of patients are referred to by the euphemism, joint venturing.

The following services are now being invested in, and then given referrals, by doctors:

- Radiology centers
- Diagnostic laboratories
- Physical rehabilitation centers
- Cardiac rehabilitation centers
- Sports medicine clinics
- Women's health centers
- Home health care and visiting nurse services
- Medical equipment leasing and sale companies
- Radiation therapy centers
- Hospital services and even hospitals themselves
- Same-day surgery centers

The situation has become so blatant, and doctors have become so desperate to increase their incomes, that doctors will now walk into the office of a specialty, such as radiology, and demand a piece of the action. Dr. William Birnbaum, a radiologist in Irvine, California, said that colleagues suddenly started demanding a share of his profits. "They said they wanted a piece of the action," Dr. Birnbaum said. "They said since it was their patients they deserve some of the income." This fee-splitting procedure has been considered highly unethical throughout the history of medicine.

As the profits from these arrangements vary anywhere from 100 to 1,000 percent, there is an incentive for doctors to bend their professional judgement. Arnold Relman, editor of the *New England Journal of Medicine*, said, "Doctors will continue to drift toward the opinion that medicine is just a business, and patients are theirs to be bought and sold." He says this unhealthy trend will continue unless these deals are outlawed.

There's No Longer a Free Market in Medicine

Dr. Relman believes that this growth in kickback ventures reflects a dramatic attitude change among physicians. Angered by the loss of income and control over patient care due to government and insurance encroachment on private practice, many physicians are fighting back in a manner the critics say breaches standards of conduct and abuses the trust of their patients.

The setting of fees by insurance companies, the corporate image given the practice of medicine by setting up so many large treatment centers, and the government's dictation of medical practice through the medicare system, make it inevitable that doctors will lose whatever sense of mission and charity they have. Many doctors see themselves, along with their patients, as victims of the system.

Few patients or employers who pay the bills are aware of these practices. But the insurance companies, whose interest is basically profit rather than care, have become aware of the situation and are reacting to it. Blue Cross/Blue Shield of Michigan has found that diagnostic laboratories owned by referring physicians charge almost double the fees of other labs and do nearly twice as many tests on the average patient. "There is no question that ownership in interest leads to more testing," said Charlotte Bartzack, a Blue Cross researcher. She found that physicians overtested pregnant women with ultrasound imaging devices, sometimes testing the women as often as once a month. There is some question as to the safety of this procedure and the result of monthly testing is not known.

I was recently made aware of the case of several oncologists getting together to finance a radiation laboratory. The gentleman who was the source of this information took a small minority ownership position to start and operate the radiation laboratory. It was financed by the three top oncologists in the area. Suddenly the demand for radiation treatment in his locale doubled, tripled, and then some.

The cross ownership of this laboratory was, to the best of the operator's knowledge, never revealed to even a single, solitary client. The operator treated the referrals, did a creditable job, and after about three years, bought the financing doctors out. So the doctors got paid by their patients, got paid again out of profits from the radiation center, and got paid a third time when they sold out at a huge profit. From the sharp increase in treatments, it's fair to assume they were prescribing radiation treatment far more than was necessary — certainly, far more than they previously thought necessary.

It is now estimated that 25 percent of physicians are holding shares in medical facilities that provide tens of billions of dollars a year in services. The transactions have spread into every aspect of medicine, even including ownership in parts of hospitals — usually the operating room or the laboratory facilities.

Even doctors who find the joint venturing unethical or distasteful are being pressured into joining the crowd. Dr. Alfred Sils, a California radiologist, led an unsuccessful fight in 1986 to outlaw these joint-venture arrangements. But last year he himself sold shares in his practice to about 40 referring physicians in order to survive. "It stinks," he said. "We held our noses and did it because if we didn't, someone else would come in here and lure our referring doctors away."

The Hypocrisy Heats Up

The American Medical Association, although not fighting these fee-splitting arrangements, has paid lip service to controlling it by requiring physicians to disclose their interest in facilities to which they refer patients. In California a state law also requires disclosure to the patient if the physician's interest in a facility amounts to five percent or $5,000. This requirement is widely ignored.

The American College of Radiology has condemned joint venturing, ostensibly to protect the interest of patients, but more likely because they are reacting against having to share their profits with other doctors. Although they are acting in their own self-interest, their statement is a model of propriety and good "civil rights" for the patients: "We have found the potential and actual abuse and exploitation of patients by unethical practices, and a flagrant disregard of physician's responsibilities to the patients so great and pervasive that these arrangements must be disallowed."

The problem has become so blatant that hucksters are now giving doctors a very direct and unequivocal pitch. One drummer for MRI units told doctors they should take advantage of the fact that their contemporaries march to the cash register. He added, "greed is a powerful motivator" and the doctors should jump on the bandwagon.

How's This for Arm-Twisting?

The situation came to a boil when a Dr. Leo Modzinski turned state's evidence against his colleagues in exchange for the government dropping charges against him.

A Michigan laboratory boasted that its limited partners received returns on their investments of between 5,000 and 7,000 percent. The Attorney General of Michigan filed criminal complaints against the lab for fraud and the payment of illegal kickbacks. Dr. Modzinski got a letter from the laboratory warning him that he would be terminated as a limited partner if his volume of lab referrals did not increase. Modzinski tried to increase his thousand-dollar initial investment but was told by the laboratory that he must generate more laboratory referrals before they would allow him to invest further. Investigators said the lab insisted that Dr. Modzinski "use lab profiles which contained unnecessary testing for many of its patients."

Unnecessary medical testing by doctors has become such a colossal drain it's now estimated that thirty-five billion dollars are wasted each year on excessive and/or unnecessary testing, not to mention the added expense of personal suffering brought about by misdiagnosis resulting from these tests.

Dr. Christopher C. Korvin reviewed 20 tests administered to 1000 hospitalized patients and found that the diagnosis of only 77 had changed as a result of the procedures done. That's a "cost-effective" level of less than eight percent.

A 1983 survey by the American Medical Association found almost half of physicians polled said that even though they were certain of their diagnosis, they did unnecessary tests because of fear of lawsuits. So the doctor alone cannot be blamed for this deplorable waste of money.

One test that analyzes the oxygen and carbon dioxide content of the blood is so inaccurate that Blue Cross/Blue Shield recommends the test to be done only in life-threatening circumstances.

Another study showed that blood pressure readings taken by doctors are inaccurate anywhere from 30 to 50 percent of the time. This means as many as one in three patients are taking powerful and dangerous drugs which are not indicated to reduce blood pressure. The elevated blood pressure, like an elevated cholesterol level, is probably the body's reaction to some pathological state and is thus a sign and not a cause of disease. Artificially lowering the blood pressure can have many disastrous effects, the primary one being a stroke — which often ends in death.

Another billion-dollar business is the twenty million electrocardiograms performed yearly. Studies have shown that about 25 percent of people diagnosed with a normal electrocardiogram, but who have symptoms of heart disease, have a heart attack. The opposite is also true in that many electrocardiograms labelled abnormal, especially in women, are in fact normal and require no treatment. But wait. It gets worse.

Payola Medicine

Patients really get hit by traffic from *two* directions. In addition to unnecessary testing that enriches their doctors, patients also have to worry about their doctors prescribing drugs because of incentives from drug companies to do so.

Do doctors really take bribes from drug companies? Sure they do. They always have. But the payola has become more blatant and expensive in recent years.

Ayerst Laboratories gives free airline tickets to faraway places to doctors who prescribe their drug,

Inderal, to 50 patients. The doctor has to fill out a form for each patient (to keep him honest). The company claims that the system uncovers medically important data. (Like which golf club the doc uses on a 75-yard approach shot.)

This drug, incidentally, causes sexual problems in practically all males taking it.

Other drug companies give all-expense-paid trips to fancy California resorts with oceanfront rooms costing $310 a night just to have the doctor hear a drug pitch by a scientist who is also handsomely paid. That's medical science?

As one company rep put it, The docs like to be stroked. Any doctor who accepts such bribery deserves to be stroked by a cat-o'-nine-tails, some would say.

There are serious questions raised by all this. How can you determine whether or not you really need that test? And is your doctor rightfully "just making sure," or is he wrongfully making a buck? And honestly, how can a doctor really be objective about prescribing a drug when the only difference (to him) is that prescribing one drug will possibly alleviate the symptoms and garner him a trip to the Bahamas — and prescribing another drug will possibly just cure the patient?

Action to Take:

Your best course of action in the face of tests your doctor requires is to ask some pointed questions. You might start with the ones posed in chapter 7 of this book. It's called "11 Questions Your Doctor Prays You Never Ask." A few which are specific to unnecessary testing are:

(1) Will this X-ray or CAT scan, if positive, have any bearing on my treatment?
(2) Will these tests contribute to my diagnosis and treatment?
(3) Would you prescribe this test for a family member with a similar problem?
(4) [For a hospital service or procedure] Could I do just as well, and would I be just as safe, at home?
(5) [For procedures required at same-day surgery centers] Will this be cheaper than the hospital and just as safe? Are they prepared for emergencies?
(6) [For tests required in any of the centers, services, or companies listed above] Do you have a financial interest in the enterprise to which you are referring me?

The answers to these questions will give you some idea how necessary the required testing is to your proper treatment. But it will also help if you do some homework before you ever step into the doctor's office. Ask your friends and acquaintances about their doctors and the frequency of tests they prescribe. Select a doctor to begin with who is conservative in prescribing tests, who seems reasonable in the overall fees he charges, and who has a good record of solving people's health problems. I don't know if it was a doctor who first said it, but "an ounce of prevention is worth a pound of cure" applies to doctor-induced woes as well as natural ones.

Chapter 7

11 Questions Your Doctor Prays You Never Ask

Many things go unsaid when you step into your doctor's office. Most people usually assume that someone who would take the Hippocratic oath and devote his life to healing people will do right by his patients. But while it's true there are a lot of honest doctors in the country, increasingly the lure of lucre or other gains causes some to resort to unethical or irresponsible practices. Many have become involved in activities which succeed in parting patients from their money, but leave their problems virtually unchanged or worse than they were before.

The questions below may not be ones you feel comfortable asking your doctor. Some of them will deal with information the doctor feels is personal, some will seem impolite, and all of them will step on toes. But when your health is at stake, there are certain things you have a right to know. You should at least know the degree of your doctor's competence, where his loyalties lie, and whether he is giving you the most efficacious treatment for your problem.

Since it would never do for you to ask your doctor: "Are you competent" (though the answer might be interesting), these questions are designed to get you the information you need to determine whether you are being treated hippocratically. Maybe you won't want to ask them if you're just in to see the doc about an ingrown toenail. But if you're there with cancer or heart disease, you *need* to know the answers to these questions. When you do, you'll know whether you're being treated well or just being treated expensively.

1. Are there any dangerous side effects from this drug?

There are always dangers, even if they are somewhat remote. You need to know the worst possibilities, as well as the best and most likely. Remember, if something affects only 1 in 10,000 people that's 25,000 folks in the U.S. If *you* have a bad reaction to a drug, that's a reaction rate of 100 percent as far as you are concerned.

2. If insurance wasn't paying for this, would you still recommend it?

The number of unnecessary tests, needless exams, noneffective medications, unneeded surgery, etc. has jumped astronomically in this country. Why? Because of the attitude that *insurance* is paying for it. "Insurance" doesn't pay for anything, *you* pay it all. (Check your next quarterly premium.)

3. When you've recommended this procedure for other patients, how many have been cured? What happened in the other cases?

If two out of three times he's recommended something, the result has been harmful — or even of no real benefit — wouldn't you like to know it? If a blood pressure medication, for instance, will lower your pressure but shorten your life, shouldn't you know that?

4. What are the possibilities I'll improve, even if I don't follow this recommendation?

When cancer patients get better because of alternative therapies, medical science calls it spontaneous remission. Most doctors refuse to acknowledge that alternative therapies have done wonders for people. Most also dislike admitting miracles occur. But they do. Get a doctor honest enough to admit how *ignorant* modern medicine is. The diagnostic equipment at our disposal is truly miraculous but the therapy offered is often worse than the disease.

5. Have you ever been sued for malpractice? What happened?

It's easy to understand why you should ask these questions and why your doctor may turn pale and get the shakes when you do, especially if he has lost a case. Losing a case doesn't always mean that the doctor was guilty of anything, juries being generally sympathetic toward the plaintiff in malpractice cases. But, even though malpractice cases are generally weighted against the doctor (he *never* gets a jury of *his* peers), when he is convicted of malpractice, he is usually guilty.

Most doctors get sued sometime during their career but some get sued more than others. So ask him how many times he has been sued successfully. A doctor who has been sued ten times but won all the suits is more likely to be a competent doctor than one who has been sued only twice but lost them both. This may sound like a truism but it is worth saying: A doctor who wins a malpractice case is usually innocent. A doctor who loses a case is usually guilty.

6. How much do you pay for malpractice insurance?

This question may not sound relevant to you but, if his malpractice rate is extremely high, it means one of two things. Either what he does is fraught with a lot of danger and undesirable complications, such as eye surgery and heart surgery, or he has been sued a lot and is thus rated higher than his colleagues doing similar medicine.

7. Are there any alternative therapies (homeopathic, natural, etc.) that have been successful with my problem? What is your opinion of them?

How open-minded is your doctor? Has he looked past the boundaries that modern medicine says are proper? If he gives you an honest answer of "I don't know," that's fine. But if he says "No, that's just a lot of quackery," then you might want to get a second opinion.

8. Do you have any financial interest in the lab or hospital that will perform this work? Are you on the board, own any stock, etc.?

If he gets upset you've asked, that will tell you plenty. *He* knows how often doctors have a built-in conflict of interest ... whether he'll admit it or not. A shocking number of doctors are tied in financially to the various services they use to make your diagnosis. This profit incentive tends to cause them to order unnecessary tests — the more they order, the more they make.

9. Have you accepted any gifts or commissions from a drug company such as a free vacation, tickets to the symphony, etc.?

Again, he might hate you for asking, but it happens all the time. And no doctor is going to *volunteer* to tell you he's doing it. It's not an illegal practice or the drug companies wouldn't risk it. But is it right and proper for your doctor to take what amounts to a bribe even though the drug firm assures the doctor that "there is no obligation"?

10. Would you prescribe the same treatment for a member of your family? Have you? What happened?

This will certainly make him think twice about giving you a drug that may cause serious side effects. I know of a case of a prominent doctor in Florida who always recommended chemotherapy for his cancer patients. But when *his* wife came down with breast cancer, he refused to let her take chemotherapy. "This is different," he said. Oh? Is it?

11. Do you do any research for drug companies? Are you doing any now? Am I being used for such research?

Doctors who do clinical research, i.e., test drugs on their patients, are extremely biased toward the drug and tend to downplay the observed side effects. They are usually paid by the pharmaceutical company which, the company knows, will tend to cause the investigator to want to come up with results favorable to the drug. It's also flattering to be chosen as an investigator and the company plays on the ego of the doctor, thus reinforcing the bias toward the agent being tested.

You may choose not to ask your doctor these questions, but you owe it to yourself to at least think about their implications and try (legally, and as unobtrusively as possible) to find out the answers to them through other means.

Another option may be to simply leave this leaflet with your doctor and tell him these are the questions you'd like to discuss with him. Then talk about them on your next visit.

However you do it, finding the answers to these questions may mean the difference between getting well and staying sick or, less critical, but still important, the difference between getting your money's worth and getting taken.

Conclusion

As you can see, there's more than enough bad medicine to go around. You really have to be careful if you want to avoid it, but doing so may be a matter of life and death some day for you or one of your loved ones. The suggestions and information in this report can help.

In addition, avoiding bad medicine will be much easier if you use the right doctor — and finding him is three-fourths the battle. If you can find an ethical doctor who believes in alternative medicine — and isn't in prison — you've really got a windfall. Don't spread the word about him carelessly or the FDA will have a *kristalnacht* at his office, but value and use his services. Such doctors are rare — and worth their weight in gold.

Index

Get a *Second Opinion* every month with Dr. Douglass' medical newsletter

Here's a shocker for you: Did you know that cancer, heart disease, the common cold, and a host of other "incurable" or "chronic" illnesses, are in many cases now completely reversible?

Did you know that garlic can help with certain forms of depression? That cabbage juice can cure the most stubborn, painful ulcer — almost immediately? That extra magnesium in your diet can reduce tendencies toward anxiety, obesity, and even heart palpitations?

It's true. And it's exactly the kind of helpful medicine that can help keep you out of your doctor's office. It'll help you live longer, feel better, even look younger. You can only find such invaluable advice in *Second Opinion*.

With *Second Opinion*, you'll see your doctor less ... spend a lot less money ... and be much happier and healthier while you're at it. Go ahead and subscribe today! When you do, we'll give you one of the reports or books described on the next three pages absolutely free ... you choose the one you want!

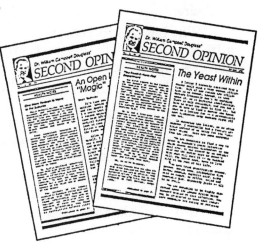

Choose your free book/report on the next three pages!

If you knew a procedure to save thousands, maybe millions of people dying from AIDS, cancer, and other dreaded killers ...

Would you cover it up?

It's unthinkable that what could be the best solution ever to stopping the world's killer diseases is being ignored, scorned, and rejected. But horrifyingly enough, that is exactly what's happening!

This remarkable procedure is called "photo-luminescence." It's a thoroughly tested, proven therapy that's performed miraculous cures around the world by stimulating the body's own immune responses. That's why it cures so many ailments — and why it's especially effective against AIDS!

Yet, 50 years ago it virtually disappeared from the halls of medicine.

Why has this incredible cure — proven effective against many ailments, from AIDS to cancer, influenza to allergies, and so much more — been ignored by the medical authorities of this country?

That's why Dr. Douglass wrote **Into the Light**. This hard-hitting, fully documented book tells the success story of photo-luminescence — who it cures, who it's helped, who covered it up and why.

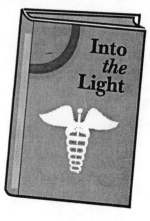

This book has everything. But most important, it tells what we need to do to make this life-saving treatment available for everyone. Get **Into the Light** now and discover the whole story for yourself.

You've got more to choose from!
See the next two pages.

The Chelation Answer

How to Prevent Hardening of the Arteries and Rejuvenate Your Cardiovascular System

By Morton Walker, DPM

Would you be relieved to hear you'll never have to worry about heart attack again — because there's an inexpensive, practically painless procedure that'll keep your heart healthy?

Would you be thrilled to hear you don't need to have a by-pass operation — because there's a safe, effective, non-surgical treatment that really works?

This life-saving treatment is available all over the country! It's called "chelation." And it has worked wonders in the lives of thousands of people.

You'll discover how it could permanently lower your blood pressure, completely reverse (or prevent) hardening of the arteries, bring back aging loved ones from senility (yes, even Alzheimer's) ... and more. Get the whole story, plus a US directory of chelation physicians, in this incredible book by Dr. Morton Walker.

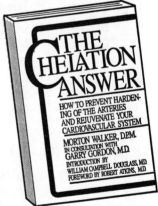

You've got more to choose from!
See the next page.

Choose one of our special reports as your free gift!

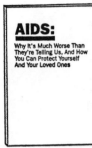

AIDS: Why It's Much Worse Than They're Telling Us, And How To Protect Yourself And Your Loved Ones

Yes, AIDS is easy to catch. No, it isn't limited to just a few groups of society. People who've never engaged in questionable behavior or come within miles of an infected needle are contracting this deadly scourge. To protect yourself, you must know the truth.

Dangerous (Legal) Drugs

If you knew what we know about the most popular prescription and over-the-counter drugs, you'd be sick. That's why Dr. Douglass wrote this shocking report. He gives you the low-down on 15 different categories of drugs: everything from painkillers and cold remedies to tranquilizers and powerful cancer drugs.

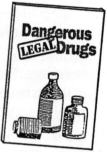

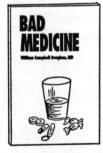

Bad Medicine

Do you really need that new prescription or that overnight stay in the hospital? In this report, Dr. Douglass reveals the common medical practices and misconceptions endangering your health. Best of all, he tells you the pointed (but very revealing!) questions your doctor prays you never ask!

Eat Your Cholesterol

Never feel guilty about what you eat again! Dr. Douglass shows you why red meat, eggs, and dairy products aren't the dietary demons we're told they are. But beware: This scientifically sound report goes against all the "common wisdom" about the foods you should eat. Read with an open mind!

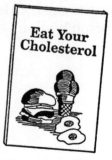

To subscribe and choose your free gift, please use the order form on the next page.

ORDER HERE

☐ **I'M SUBSCRIBING to** *Second Opinion* **at just $49 for 12 issues (cover price: $96 per year — I save 48%!).** I want to protect those I love from the health dangers the authorities aren't telling me about.... and the incredible remedies that they've scorned and ignored. This kind of information is vital to my health. Sign me up for *Second Opinion* — and don't forget to send me my free gift. The free report/book I want is

_____ .

(choose 1 title from below)

I'd like to buy the following:

Qty.	Title	Price	Amount
____	1 Year/*Second Opinion*	$49	$_____
____	Into the Light	$24.50	$_____
____	The Chelation Answer	$14.95	$_____
____	AIDS: What They're Not Telling You	$ 8.95	$_____
____	Dangerous (Legal) Drugs	$ 8.95	$_____
____	Bad Medicine	$ 8.95	$_____
____	Eat Your Cholesterol	$ 8.95	$_____

If not subscribing, add shipping/handling per order:
$2.50 first item, .50¢ each additional item $_____

TOTAL $_____

☐ My payment of $_____ is enclosed.
☐ Charge my: ☐ MasterCard ☐ Visa

Card#_____

Signature_____ Exp._____

Name_____

Address_____

City_____State_____Zip_____

Telephone_____

BADM94

Call Toll-Free
1-800-728-2288
Fax: 404-399-0815

Mail to: *Second Opinion*
P.O. Box 467939 • Atlanta, GA 31146-7939

"Love *Second Opinion!*"

— *G.B.F., Mt. Pleasant, TX*

Here are just a few good things we've
heard about Dr. William Campbell Douglass
and *Second Opinion.*

**You are indeed a "second opinion."
You are brilliant and provocative.**

— *Dr. T.M.D., Leonia, NJ*

**Your *Second Opinion* is a breath of fresh air.
Keep up the good work, and for God's sake,
continue bowing to no one.**

— *R.V.F., Ph.D., Santa Barbara, CA*

**I am glad to find someone,
especially an actual medical doctor,
who is saying what I have suspected
for some time.**

— *W.M.M., Ashland, VA*

**Frankly, I trust your judgment.
I base many of the questions I ask
my family physician on information I get
from your superb newsletter.**

— *J.M., Jacksonville, FL*

William Campbell Douglass, MD graduated from the
University of Rochester, the Miami School of Medicine, and
the Naval School of Aviation and Space Medicine. He has been
named the National Health Federation's "Doctor of the Year."

Dr. Douglass is a popular speaker who has appeared on
radio and television hundreds of times over the years. The
author of five books and numerous articles, he also travels
widely. A former practicing physician who in the past operated
clinics on three continents, Dr. Douglass is now editor-in-chief
of the alternative medicine newsletter *Second Opinion.*

ORDER HERE

☐ **I'M SUBSCRIBING** to *Second Opinion* at just $49 for 12 issues (cover price: $96 per year — I save 48%!). I want to protect those I love from the health dangers the authorities aren't telling me about ... and the incredible remedies that they've scorned and ignored. This kind of information is vital to my health. Sign me up for *Second Opinion* — and don't forget to send me my free gift. The free report/book I want is

_____.

(choose 1 title from below)

I'd like to buy the following:

Qty.	Title	Price	Amount
____	1 Year/*Second Opinion*	$49	$_____
____	Into the Light	$24.50	$_____
____	The Chelation Answer	$14.95	$_____
____	AIDS: What They're Not Telling You	$ 8.95	$_____
____	Dangerous (Legal) Drugs	$ 8.95	$_____
____	Bad Medicine	$ 8.95	$_____
____	Eat Your Cholesterol	$ 8.95	$_____

If not subscribing, add shipping/handling per order: $2.50 first item, .50¢ each additional item $_____

TOTAL $_____

☐ My payment of $_____ is enclosed.
☐ Charge my: ☐ MasterCard ☐ Visa

Card#_____

Signature_____ Exp._____

Name _____

Address_____

City_____State_____Zip_____

Telephone_____

BADM94

Call Toll-Free
1-800-728-2288
Fax: 404-399-0815

Mail to: *Second Opinion*
P.O. Box 467939 • Atlanta, GA 31146-7939

"Love Second Opinion!"

— G.B.F., Mt. Pleasant, TX

Here are just a few good things we've
heard about Dr. William Campbell Douglass
and *Second Opinion*.

**You are indeed a "second opinion."
You are brilliant and provocative.**

— Dr. T.M.D., Leonia, NJ

**Your *Second Opinion* is a breath of fresh air.
Keep up the good work, and for God's sake,
continue bowing to no one.**

— R.V.F., Ph.D., Santa Barbara, CA

**I am glad to find someone,
especially an actual medical doctor,
who is saying what I have suspected
for some time.**

— W.M.M., Ashland, VA

**Frankly, I trust your judgment.
I base many of the questions I ask
my family physician on information I get
from your superb newsletter.**

— J.M., Jacksonville, FL

William Campbell Douglass, MD graduated from the
University of Rochester, the Miami School of Medicine, and
the Naval School of Aviation and Space Medicine. He has been
named the National Health Federation's "Doctor of the Year."

Dr. Douglass is a popular speaker who has appeared on
radio and television hundreds of times over the years. The
author of five books and numerous articles, he also travels
widely. A former practicing physician who in the past operated
clinics on three continents, Dr. Douglass is now editor-in-chief
of the alternative medicine newsletter *Second Opinion*.

ORDER HERE

☐ **I'M SUBSCRIBING** to *Second Opinion* at just $49 for 12 issues (cover price: $96 per year — I save 48%!). I want to protect those I love from the health dangers the authorities aren't telling me about ... and the incredible remedies that they've scorned and ignored. This kind of information is vital to my health. Sign me up for *Second Opinion* — and don't forget to send me my free gift. The free report/book I want is

_____.

(choose 1 title from below)

I'd like to buy the following:

Qty.	Title	Price	Amount
____	1 Year/*Second Opinion*	$49	$_____
____	Into the Light	$24.50	$_____
____	The Chelation Answer	$14.95	$_____
____	AIDS: What They're Not Telling You	$ 8.95	$_____
____	Dangerous (Legal) Drugs	$ 8.95	$_____
____	Bad Medicine	$ 8.95	$_____
____	Eat Your Cholesterol	$ 8.95	$_____

If not subscribing, add shipping/handling per order: $2.50 first item, .50¢ each additional item $_____

TOTAL $_____

☐ My payment of $_____ is enclosed.
☐ Charge my: ☐ MasterCard ☐ Visa

Card#_____

Signature_____ Exp._____

Name _____
Address_____
City_____ State_____ Zip_____
Telephone_____

BADM94

Call Toll-Free
1-800-728-2288
Fax: 404-399-0815

Mail to: *Second Opinion*
P.O. Box 467939 • Atlanta, GA 31146-7939

"Love *Second Opinion!*"

— G.B.F., Mt. Pleasant, TX

Here are just a few good things we've heard about Dr. William Campbell Douglass and *Second Opinion.*

You are indeed a "second opinion." You are brilliant and provocative.

— Dr. T.M.D., Leonia, NJ

Your *Second Opinion* is a breath of fresh air. Keep up the good work, and for God's sake, continue bowing to no one.

— R.V.F., Ph.D., Santa Barbara, CA

I am glad to find someone, especially an actual medical doctor, who is saying what I have suspected for some time.

— W.M.M., Ashland, VA

Frankly, I trust your judgment. I base many of the questions I ask my family physician on information I get from your superb newsletter.

— J.M., Jacksonville, FL

William Campbell Douglass, MD graduated from the University of Rochester, the Miami School of Medicine, and the Naval School of Aviation and Space Medicine. He has been named the National Health Federation's "Doctor of the Year."

Dr. Douglass is a popular speaker who has appeared on radio and television hundreds of times over the years. The author of five books and numerous articles, he also travels widely. A former practicing physician who in the past operated clinics on three continents, Dr. Douglass is now editor-in-chief of the alternative medicine newsletter *Second Opinion.*

ORDER HERE

☐ **I'M SUBSCRIBING** to *Second Opinion* at just $49 for 12 issues (cover price: $96 per year — I save 48%!). I want to protect those I love from the health dangers the authorities aren't telling me about... and the incredible remedies that they've scorned and ignored. This kind of information is vital to my health. Sign me up for *Second Opinion* — and don't forget to send me my free gift. The free report/book I want is

_____.

(choose 1 title from below)

I'd like to buy the following:

Qty.	Title	Price	Amount
____	1 Year/*Second Opinion*	$49	$_____
____	Into the Light	$24.50	$_____
____	The Chelation Answer	$14.95	$_____
____	AIDS: What They're Not Telling You	$ 8.95	$_____
____	Dangerous (Legal) Drugs	$ 8.95	$_____
____	Bad Medicine	$ 8.95	$_____
____	Eat Your Cholesterol	$ 8.95	$_____

If not subscribing, add shipping/handling per order: $2.50 first item, .50¢ each additional item $_____

TOTAL $_____

☐ My payment of $_____ is enclosed.
☐ Charge my: ☐ MasterCard ☐ Visa

Card#_____

Signature_____ Exp._____

Name_____
Address_____
City_____State_____Zip_____
Telephone_____

BADM94

Call Toll-Free
1-800-728-2288
Fax: 404-399-0815

Mail to: *Second Opinion*
P.O. Box 467939 • Atlanta, GA 31146-7939

"Love *Second Opinion!*"

— *G.B.F., Mt. Pleasant, TX*

Here are just a few good things we've
heard about Dr. William Campbell Douglass
and *Second Opinion.*

You are indeed a "second opinion."
You are brilliant and provocative.

— *Dr. T.M.D., Leonia, NJ*

Your *Second Opinion* is a breath of fresh air.
Keep up the good work, and for God's sake,
continue bowing to no one.

— *R.V.F., Ph.D., Santa Barbara, CA*

I am glad to find someone,
especially an actual medical doctor,
who is saying what I have suspected
for some time.

— *W.M.M., Ashland, VA*

Frankly, I trust your judgment.
I base many of the questions I ask
my family physician on information I get
from your superb newsletter.

— *J.M., Jacksonville, FL*

William Campbell Douglass, MD graduated from the
University of Rochester, the Miami School of Medicine, and
the Naval School of Aviation and Space Medicine. He has been
named the National Health Federation's "Doctor of the Year."

Dr. Douglass is a popular speaker who has appeared on
radio and television hundreds of times over the years. The
author of five books and numerous articles, he also travels
widely. A former practicing physician who in the past operated
clinics on three continents, Dr. Douglass is now editor-in-chief
of the alternative medicine newsletter *Second Opinion*.